A Yogi's Guide to Yoga

By: Brianne Moran, a teenage yogi

A Yogi's
Guide to Yoga

Copyright ©2018
Brianne Moran

Introduction

You hear people say, meditation is good for the mind and body, that it can heal and strengthen your body, and that it teaches you to connect with yourself. Even so, many still say yoga is just for hippies, it's not real exercise, and it's a scam. They rail against it and say that all it really is just stretching for an hour or so. With all of this confusion and disagreement, it is here that my journey begins.

 Before I reached 3 years of age, I had already suffered from 13 ear infections. Having two sets of tubes in my ears, as well as an adenoidectomy and tonsillectomy, my pediatrician visits grew to become a familiar routine. People would usually call it a sympathetical or pity 'wow' experience, though the expericine was far more traumatic! As I grew more sickly, these culminated health issues threw off my balance to walk properly; resulting in long term conditions and problems in walking and running.

Due to my condition, at an early age when kids are the most active, I had casts and braces on my legs at three different times. While kids in pre-k were sitting in circles in class and running around the playground, I had to get a special staircase so I can walk at my own pace and my mom had to carry me to different places. The casts were on both of my legs and made walking around hard, and even harder to do the things I wanted to do. Physical therapy was a big milestone in my recovery. I took a big leap from struggling to walk to joining a soccer and swim team. I took physical therapy at children's specialized hospital in Mountainside, New Jersey. My physical therapist was also a yoga instructor. My instructor helped me using different yoga techniques to assist in the recovery of the bone misplacement in my leg. During physical therapy, we would always start off with yoga. Using yoga made my recovery faster than what I saw in other children. Many kids and adults sympathised with me, thinking the infections and physical therapy would give me trauma, but I did not. I grew from these experiences and they made me the person I am today. . After taking the casts off, I was able to joined swim teams and do kickboxing and all the other things kids love to do.

After physical therapy, I felt that yoga was beneficial to keep in my life. As I continued to practice yoga, I discovered yoga not only helped with the physical aspect of my life, but my mental state as well. My academics were very strong. I was fortunate enough to be into Honors classes, which created lots of stress. On top of that, because of my dad's job, I constantly moved. This lead to even more anxiety. I tried multiple methods to lowering stress levels. The most effective method I noticed was yoga. It helped so much that my anxiety levels went down. The more I practiced, the more I could concentrate & focus. This method helped me focus in school and get good grades without stressing out. The anxiety that I would have everyday would go down. I realised that it was a great method to use when I was stressed and needed help concentrating.

Looking back, I wished I knew the things then that I now know as a teenager. All those years of casts on and off could have been avoided and those long periods of physical therapy could have been shortened through more yoga!. That's why I am writing this book, to show people that are in the same situation , that there are alternatives to standard western medicine. It's a given that people struggle in life; whether it is to find peace in their own bodies,or a battle with anxiety, cancer or other combatants we may face in the future.

People that practice yoga know the wonders of doing meditation. It has helped people boost their immune system and negate other deficiencies in their lives. This book will help those looking to get the most out of their lives. Yoga can even help with various diseases.

If you are willing to keep an open mind, I will show through this book various studies and milestones that were made through yoga and mediation.

Yoga has always had a bad image. This image is perpetrated by people who do not perform it properly. Many don't even see the little changes that happens with their body and their lives. I really feel through my trial and error my life change. I never really practiced self care until I started doing yoga and fell in love with it. Yoga is a time where you can really connect with yourself on a spiritual level and start your journey of finding yourself. It can also help your blood flow, breathing fluctuations, and your muscles. As you read, you will learn how taking care of your body does not always mean exercising and drinking smoothies and eating salads. It also has to do with learning to love your body, and connecting yourself spiritually is also part of taking care of it. There will be stories of people discovering a new way to health and self discovery.

The yoga philosophy

There are eight major chakras, each chakra represent each centre of your body that releases energy. Sushumna Nadi is your energy pathway, the chakras lie on these pathways. What yoga does to these pathways is unblocks them and cleanse your energetic body. Along with this, there are levels or layers to each represents us spiritually and our existence called Koshas. This may sound like a multiple of information, however, it is very easy to understand in the process of meditation, This is only the chip of the iceberg, so let's dig deeper

Muladhara chakra (base or root chakra)

This chakra is associated with security, being close to earth and survival. It is known as the element of earth and the colour association is red. The placement is at the base of the spine. The chakra is surrounded by health, so to keep our awareness and neuter to this chakra it is beneficial to do exercise. For example, jumping, running, and dancing are good to do to keep this chakra healthy. This chakra is meant to create security and an enjoyable place in life. The message or mantra to be said is "I exist" and to live your life proudly.

Svadhisthana Chakra (Sacral Chakra)

The chakra Svadhisthana is known for the desire for pleasure and sensuality. The colour is orange and the element is associated with water. The location is the lower abdomen, so typically belly-dancing, loving, and yoga will help improve the function of this.

"This chakra says, "I desire". Live your passion, whatever that may be. What are your dreams? How do you desire to live? Claim your dreams and go out and make them a reality – give birth to your dreams." - Iarp. "Chakra Basics: Learn What Chakras are and their Energetic Properties." IARP, IARP, 29 Dec. 2016, iarp.org/chakra-basics/.

Manipura chakra (Between the navel and solar plexus)

The colour for this chakra is yellow, a bright colour to show the overbearing solar plexus chakra. This means that this chakra is not balanced with the other ones and your energy is solely focused. The element is fire and is related to the power in the world. The term 'fire in your belly' is derived from this. This can become an obsessive control if not controlled, the message is also "I control". It can become good or bad, if healthy it can control your destiny and accomplished goals.

Anahata chakra (heart)

The element that goes with this chakra is air and relates to love and compassion. The colour is green and it's at the heart centre for the representation of love. This goes with healthy relationships with pets, family, and even a love for the beauty of nature help this chakra. The message is "I love"

"Let your heart energy flow freely in and out. Be open to receiving the love that is available to you now, the free-flowing love that is your birthright. Sense your Reiki family around the world – feel the great love that you all share and that you selflessly emanate from this world."

-Iarp. "Chakra Basics: Learn What Chakras are and their Energetic Properties." IARP, 29 Dec. 2016, iarp.org/chakra-basics/.

Vishuddhi chakra (throat)

The chakra is the communication centre to speak honesty and truth, the colour is blue and the element is sound. When this chakra is healthy you can speak with courage and have the power to ask for what you need. Practice such as singing, chanting, and breathing exercises help improve the health of Vishuddhi. The message for this chakra is "I express".

Ajna chakra (third eye)

The chakra of the third eye has the properties of awareness, guidance, intuition, and insight. The colour for this chakra is represented in indigo, it is located in between the eyebrows. The unique element of physic power on your side, using meditation and visualization practices create the healthy flow. The mantra is "I am the witness"

Sahasrara Chakra (crown)

The representation of spiritual connection is located on the top of the head or crown. The colour that is used mostly by Reiki practitioners is the colour of the crown which is violet or the colour violet-white light. Bliss, union, and the knowledge of being one with all are part of Sahasrara. With the frequency of cosmic consciousness and peace at your side it will help you connect more with yourself and spirit. The message is "I am that I am"

Bindu chakra (beneath the cowlick)

Unlike the others, this chakras colour is transparent or colourless. It is known as the nectar of immortality with the mantra being "I am immortal". Consciousness is the main focus and the symbol is a crescent moon which is supposed to hold the nectar. With qualities of youthfulness, health, healing, harmony, and clarity. It helps calm your emotion and help eyesight. To practice this chakra is to have the experience of the other chakras, making this chakra known as the end of your journey. It involves a great amount of advance meditation and practice.

The three main Nadis

The word Nadi means flow, this is where the life force or "prana" circulate. Of the fourteen principal Nadis, these three are known to be the most important. To explain the three, I will be talking about the words masculine and feminine. It is not in the sense of sex but as more of traits inside of each Nadi. The yoga that is used with the thought of nadis is Kundalini yoga. "The technique of Kundalini Yoga consists in using Prana (the vital air), guiding its circulatory movement through Ida and Pingala down to the base of the spine into space where Kundalini lies coiled. The vital energies of the opposite forces circulating in Ida and

Pingala will be unified and Shakti Kundalini will then awaken and rise up Sushumna, energizing the seven chakras."

-Harish Johari. " Chakras: Energy Centers of Transformation ." Tantra Kundalini, Destiny Books, a division of Inner Traditions International, Rochester, www.tantra-kundalini.com/nadis.htm

Sushumna- The central channel, associated with the river Saraswati. Inside this channel, there are three smaller channels called Vajra, Chitrini and Brahma. The practice of Kundalini makes the movement of energy upwards running up the body from below Muladhara chakra to the crown of the head.

Ida- This is the left channel, connecting to the left nostril. It is associated with femininity and the colour white. Correlated with cold, the moon, and the river Ganga.

Pingala- The opposite of Ida, it is connected to the right channel and right nostril. Associated with masculinity, hot, the sun, and correlated with the colour red. Both Ida and Pingala were originated in Muladhara.

Koshas

Koshas are used to be a great guide to the body to visually and mentally sense what you are benefiting from when doing yoga. You can get stuck in each layer which makes you pay less attention to the others and hurts the potential to be to your fullest. Koshas are dimensions, from the dimension of your physical body to the spiritual centre. They each have energy and move at different speeds, they interact with each other, and are the holders of our energy.

Annamaya Kosha (The earth element):

It is the first layer. The physical form is the densest of them all, it contains all the bones and organs. The first layer also has the lowest vibration, to keep the atoms making up your body together. The word anna derives from the word food, this is because this layer is made up of what we eat. To get stuck in this layer is to become obsessive about your body image and focus on the way you look at an anxiety driven stage.

Pranamaya Kosha (fire and water elements):

The second layer is the energy dimension is consists of the life source that moves through the nadis. It consists of the literal breath, the flow of blood; carries impulses to the nerves, brain, and back. What makes these functions are the five pranas -prana means energy- called: Prana, Apana, Udana, Samana, and Vyana. Without them, the body will become lifeless and unable to think and move. Prana goes throughout different sheaths using nadis along with different energy types like mental and psychic. This allows us to grow and develop the more we age, both mentally and physically.

Manamaya kosha (air and space elements):

The third kosha is about the dimension of mentality, the word mana means mind. It is inclusive of our thoughts, feelings, mind, and our emotions. We commonly use the animal monkey to show an example of this dimension. This is because we view the world with what gives us pleasure and hate or known as raga and dvesha. Raga means desire and dvesha means hate, to the most simplified version of it, we experience pain and pleasure which makes us respond with either positive or negative emotion. To get stuck at this level is to get lost in your thoughts or the 'mental withdrawing of the senses'. Practices such as pranayama and pratyahara yoga are very effective.

This layer focuses on the three levels of consciousness. Consciousness, by definition, is about having a connection with the outer world through the senses. The mind functions on three levels:

• Conscious: the connection of the mind to the outer world through the brain.

• Subconscious: the mind assortment of all your memories

• Unconscious mind: Your 'Real Self' or known as the 'Atman'

Vijnanamaya Kosha (wisdom)

Unlike the other mental kosha, there is no physical form. This kosha correlates with higher levels of consciousness, this sheath includes becoming aware that the mind and body are lost.   Vijnana means subtle wisdom and knowledge, trying to reach an intuitive level of knowledge. In this dimension, it incorporates our knowledge of self-awareness, decision making and judgement. It is the established higher mind, even so, this higher mind goes toward the soul seeking truth and searching for the eternal centre of consciousness. Vijnanamaya Kosha, with the help of nadis, makes the connection of the conscious mind to the higher and universal mind. To practice this kosha, it is best to practice the meditation type called Dharana. You can also do dhyana which is the mental focus on an object and dhyana, which is another way to meditate. These inner inculcations moves us closer to our goal to channel our focus towards a level of consciousness

Anandamaya Kosha (element of space)

The definition of the word Ananda comes from the word bliss. The last layer is the spiritual or true form of the body, this is where the body becomes one with the 'divine spark' or the soul. The kosha Anandamaya is connected with the superconscious mind. To awaken the sense of connection to all, it is when the higher mind combines with the super conscious or unconscious mind. This has the highest level of vibration and the thinnest, opposite of the first and densest layer. This is the layer of realization of the self or god, which you reach liberation or 'Mukti'. Not many people go to this level, mostly saints and realized souls.

Finding yourself through yoga

Self discovery does not always seem like a important topic in people daily lives. The journey of self discovery is long and can last almost your whole life, I'm still on the journey. A part of my

 journey is when I struggled with self awareness for my multiple heritages. I became grateful to be exposed to these cultures and know that I am more culturally aware then most of my peers growing up. My Native American culture taught me to use meditation to find self awareness. I would meditate at home and with my family, it help me find happiness and peace with my mind and body. My African American heritage taught me that yoga can be used to help your spirituality. Finding spirituality with my family means finding faith and practicing Christianity and putting it into yoga. Along with my Italian heritage that found that yoga to help with the mind and soul. Which I found great results in with my life

Tibetan Buddhist Meditation for Concentration

This form of meditation is used to help with concentration abilities, during the practice the body becomes increasingly aware on how it functions and how scattered brain we are. It involves keeping a mental image of either a Buddha or anything you would like it to be. This method does not always work with everyone, some have peace of mind while others can find it terribly uncomfortable. This method is for a limited few but it is always fun to try it out.

To do this meditation it is vital to focus on your own breath, to bring awareness to your breath is the objective to doing with meditation. As you are doing this method, it is important to try to focus the movement of your breath. Using mental images of how your movements are used makes it easier for some, while focusing on a patterent can help with others.

If focusing on breathing is hard, another technique is to focus on the mind itself. Using mindfulness to focus on the object in your head or concentrating on the beat of your breath can make it easier too. Again, this method does not work for everyone so always stop if it makes you uncomfortable. Many try to continue even if it makes them uncomfortable and the more they practice the worse it gets. Try to relax into it and slowly it will bring self awareness.

Sufi meditation for self discovery

Just like how buddhist meditation was for concentration, Sufi meditation is used for self discovery and the heart chakra. An article from Sufism Journal states, " In Sufi meditation, a seeker will learn how to take hold of his or her energies from all these lines of communication and collect them from the outside to direct them to the center of the heart." After using this type of meditation, it will bring awareness to yourself and finding your central point. To practice this type of meditation , it is important to try to concentrate all your energy into your heart. Doing this requires long periods of practice people that are willing to do this will notice how bringing yourself into awareness and how mentally improved you will feel. This form of meditation will bring the energy that you put into the world back into your heart. Since there are steps to meditation, there are ways to make this easier to practice. For example, if I know that I have a busy day ahead of me, I would practice this method in my room before I would get dressed. This type of meditation is really useful in the morning, it makes your whole day feeling like you have room for more energy. This is one type of meditation that I use more than others because I run out of energy during the end of the day and using this can really give you more awareness.

Using meditation to help anxiety

Meditation can really be anything you want it to be, simple breathing meditation to trying to find inner peace. The main reason why I got into meditation was to help with my anxiety, I would meditate during school and every morning and night. Even small five minute ones could change your entire day.

Mantras

The meditation I do is small but has a great impact. To help with anxiety, what I had noticed that would help was reciting mantras. Mantras are small phrases or words that will be your small goal for that day. For example, if you have a busy day before doing work, reciting words like 'calm', 'peace', or even saying 'I will do all my work today is a good start'. When I start meditating in the morning I recite the words 'I am enough', because I always have a tendency to put my expectations for myself higher than anything I can ever reach. Mantras can be any words of comfort or goals.

Hand positions (Mudras)

There are many ways to rest your hands on your knees, there are different ones that can help with multiple types of meditation. The three types that I do are excellent for breathing and self awareness. One of them is called Dhyana Mudra, it is the most basic and simple to learn and is great for beginners. The right hand rest on top of the left with the two thumbs touching each other. It is very comfortable and is used mostly in buddhist meditation. The next type is for calmness and it is called the Vayu Mudra, it is where you put the the point of your index finger and let your thumb hug around it. This is good for meditation to find inner peace and to help with stress, and also for people with hyperactive minds. ANother type of Mudra is one that I use that was something I discovered while attending a yoga camp, this type is good for breathing, and people that struggle with breathing. First place your thumb to your closest finger, then every short inhale move your thumb to the next finger. When you reach the pinky, go in reverse and move your finger for every short exhale. Keep repeating this movement during your practice. This can be useful for people that loses their breath easily or for people that are stressful.

Breathing

Last and certainly not least, is breathing. Breathing is the most important thing in meditation, it can either make or break your practice. It is also the most flexible technique in your practice. For calming the senses, longer breaths are more important. The longer the breaths you can take while being comfortable, the more peaceful you will feel. The more stress you feel the more you take shorter breaths, monitor your breaths, and may even over breathe. This can also be related to meditation and yoga, that is why breathing can quickly ruin the experience. With practicing meditation longer, breathing will become easier. The most vital breathing technique can be up to you! Everyone learns differently and will breathe differently too. You can keep count of the seconds, for example inhale and exhale every ten seconds. Keeping a beat in your head to even blinking to the beat of your lungs, all of these techniques are really important.

Meditation can help everyone of all ages and it is never too late to start. Just doing it three minutes a day can help you for your whole entire day. Small changes like these can help you on your track to a more positive lifestyle.

Hot yoga

There are different ways to deal with your depression and anxiety and one such way is through hot yoga. Yoga is a great factor to mental health and can help calm nerves and settle minds. Hot yoga is not only to help with weight loss, but can also help the psyche. I practice hot yoga about twice a week and I noticed improvements in my mental well-being and I have more energy. I feel like it's just as important as meditation and needs to be bring into awareness for beginners in yoga. [1]Publications, Harvard Health. "Yoga for anxiety and depression." Harvard Health Letter, states that yoga lowers physiological and physical tension, such as reducing heart rate, lowering blood pressure, and easing respiration. "Yoga appears to modulate stress response systems," which means that yoga can be an effective reducer to stress and mood swings.

---

[1] Publications, Harvard Health. "Yoga for anxiety and depression." Harvard Health, Harvard Medical school, Apr. 2009, www.health.harvard.edu/mind-and-mood/yoga-for-anxiety-and-depression. Accessed 17 Sept. 2017.

Different roles in Hot Yoga:

I will be going over different types of benefits in hot yoga and the reaction to the body when doing this practice. Hot yoga has different levels of difficulty; hotter rooms are expected for more experienced people in yoga, it's always good to start out with the cooler rooms. I will be going over Bikram and Hot Vinyasa, some of the more common ones and how it detoxifies and flush your body of toxins.

Bikram Yoga

Bikram yoga is one of the best yoga for depression, anxiety, mood swings, and menstrual cycles. This form of yoga is much harder than yoga like Vinyasa. The room will most likely be 105 degree fahrenheit, holding poses longer. The goal of this is to increase flexibility and lower anxiety and stiffness in the body.

Physical improvements

There has been great improvements in the body such as lowering blood pressure, back pain, and cholesterol. Bikram yoga has helped show improvements in bodies with hypertension, it is also a great natural alternative to medication. First your blood pressure will peak a little bit higher, than it will start a natural decrease returning to normal levels. This takes time and dedication for hot yoga to work, after a year or so you will see improvements. Even so, always remember to consult your doctor first hand if you have any risk factors and always take your time.

Bikram yoga is also a natural remedy to nerve and back pain, each pose and each position is designed for your back to relax and make your back comfortable. In an article named [2]"Bikram Yoga and Back Pain" it states that the author described that her back pain has been going on for awhile and that when she was doing yoga, the more she did it, the faster she saw recovery. She states, "Now, eleven years out from the initial bad spell, I live a free, active life….There are no yoga poses that I skip or avoid. I haven't thrown out my back since 2004." Yoga has helped many

---

[2] By Portsmouth. "Bikram Yoga and Back Pain." *Bikram Yoga Portsmouth*, Portsmouth wordpress, 15 May 2014, byportsmouth.wordpress.com/2014/03/21/bikram-yoga-and-back-pain/. Accessed 17 Sept. 2017.

people with similar problems as hers.

Cholesterol is another big affect to the body during Bikram. During the poses in Bikram, it allows the body to have easy blood flow as well as clean the arteries and with long time commitment, you can really see a big improvement.

Mental improvements

Stress can play a grand role in your journey into Bikram yoga, along with depression and sleep problems.

Stress is a constant part of your life, that is why it is important to find time to relive it, Bikram yoga is one example of a beautiful reliever. Bikram forces yourself to really focus on your body and how mentally relaxed you feel in that present moment. It calms the body and lifts the weight of pressure off your shoulders.

Depression can also be linked to problems sleeping, and yoga has a big impact on both depression and insomnia. It may be surprising to find out that yoga is heavily linked to impacting sleep physiology. It's has shown to help people with sleep disorders, making even the most nocturnal night-owls recover their sleep pattern. Depression is one of the most growing mood disorders in north america, it affects millions of adults along with children. Bikram yoga has shown to be a natural anti-depression. In the same article by Harvard Health "Yoga for anxiety and depression", researchers of Harvard conducted an experiment with people that have mental illness and how yoga affects their mental health and state of mind. They stated, "At the end of three months, women in the yoga group reported improvements in perceived stress, depression, anxiety, energy, fatigue, and well-being. Depression scores improved by 50%, anxiety scores by 30%, and overall well-being scores by 65%. Initial complaints of headaches, back pain, and poor sleep quality also resolved much more often in the yoga group than in the control group." This shows how doing yoga can improve the way our brain functions and the improvement of Bikram yoga has on us.

The same article, "Bikram Yoga and back pain", also

has stated, "I recommend Bikram Yoga because it is a therapeutic series and it works. It was scientifically designed to work the entire body and you don't have to worry if the flow your teacher designed today will be right for you." Bikram can be for anyone, along with the amazing natural benefits it is a great type of hot yoga to practice.

Hot Vinyasa

On the opposing end of Bikram yoga, Hot Vinyasa includes more movement into your practice. Meaning there is a little more difficulty in concentration and steadiness but with this practice it is easy to understand and get used too very quickly. Such as Bikram yoga, it has many great long term benefits. It has been shown to help those with asthma, cardiovascular disease, Carpal tunnel disease, and migraines. Along with mental complications such as, anxiety disorders, depression, and stress and tension.

Mental benefits include helping with depression and tension in the body and mind. Like bikram yoga, it has almost the same natural benefits. Along with physical prosperities which include helping the heart, breathing, and the head.

Hot yoga can be beneficial to anyone, even if it is hard to

get strayed into yoga and sometimes a big struggle.

Overcoming that hurdle can lead to have a long and healthy

life.

Interview and in-depth understanding of yoga

I was able to interview Robin Dyon, she is a yoga instructor at decatur yoga. I wanted to interview someone who has been practicing yoga for years.

What made you become a yoga instructor?

"I became a yoga instructor because I was practicing yoga and I fell in love with yoga, I've been doing it for so long at Decatur with so many good teachers it just seemed like a natural progression for me. I was a former dancer, athlete, and I loved the practice and the teachings. It just became a natural progression that I become a teacher, I have been teaching for five years."

Is there any kind of self awareness that goes into meditation and yoga?

"Oh my god yes! That's all yoga and meditation really is, is self awareness because yoga makes you a better version of you and the only way to become a better version of yourself is to be aware of what you do, how you react, and who you are in the world. This is how you can be a better person and a better person for people.”

What benefits have you seen in yoga for others and yourself?

“Well for me-like you said self awareness- it keeps you in check. Being Mindful, being aware of what you say and what you do and how it has an effect on others. Yoga for me; it just made me try to be thoughtful, more patient, kinder, and a better listener. Things that you want to be, helps you be that. Because yoga is just about you and your body and you breathe. Your spending time with yourself. That's the most wonderful thing about yoga,that there's no way your thinking about anything else then what's going on in that moment then your body and your breathe. It's really hard too. And the thing thing that I love about meditation, is that what it does physically for you, is opens you up, creates space; gets some of the 'kinks' out so you can sit deeper in your meditation and you can work deeper and better into your meditation so it's basically just sitting with yourself. It just helps you tolerate yourself"

-Yoga shows many benefits after you are done, it brings to you a inner peace and relaxation that also makes your senses more aware of your actions and choices you do. It brings awareness to how you react to others and the way they react to you. Yoga helps calm and resets your systems, so when you go out into the busy and stressful world you almost view it in a different sense. This helps make you think and act more positively due to the lack of stress that you once entered in the yoga room with.

What have you seen help people with anxiety and depression with yoga?

"I'm glad that you're asking me that because I'm an example of that. My daughter, eighteen years ago, when I gave birth to her I got postpartum depression and it's basically a chemical imbalance. I was a pretty...adjusted person I didn't really feel bad, I didn't really struggle. I was more anxious but I handled it, after I had my daughter Ruby, I just noticed that I was not happy, I was more anxious than ever, I couldn't really function like I used to. So I got on medication and it was numbing me and I hated it. Then I, kinda let my yoga practice fall to the waist-side. When I was pregnant with Rub, I just didn't have the time and I really didn't have the desire because I started to get depressed. And my husband gave me a gift certificate to decatur yoga fourteen years ago and it was for five classes. They only taught Bikram, 90 minutes of Bikram than any other style so it was really hard. When I took the first class, I thought I was connecting with the people there. I noticed that I felt better and I thought,'Well I'm going to try this thirty-day yoga challenge and not take my meds' and see if yoga did the same thing that my meds did. And it did, because when your depressed, it's chemical-your imbalanced. What happens when you do yoga? You get calmer, more balanced, ao it really is a natural drug"

-As a person with anxiety and depression, I have also felt the difference in my mental state when I was practicing yoga and meditation. I noticed my mood swings become shorter and not as harsh, I truly felt a difference in how I felt during long periods of doing yoga and meditating. Many people do yoga for the physical benefits but laying underneath all the visions of getting healthy, there is a beautiful utopia of mental aspects.

What are your best tips for beginners and people trying out yoga?

I say the most important thing is to not look around and compare themselves to everyone else. Classes are great because you can see what's going on and you have visual, community, and support, especially when you can hear everyone's breathe. But, a lot of people are insecure because they can't do poses or struggle to keep up. The most important thing I say to somebody new is, 'Don't feel like you have to keep up the shapes or do what everyone else is doing. You go in there and just see what it feels like'. Listen to your breathe, take child's pose if you need to. Know and respect where your at and then see where that goes.

What I say to new struggling people is 'What are you good at?' at somebody and they will say something like, 'Well I'm a doctor I'm good at saving people.' Well, how many years did it get you there? You just got to be patient. Especially with younger kids, they need to see the immediacy of things. Yoga is not going to do that it's the opposite of it."

- The hardest part of getting into anything, is starting it. There is always stories of how many people do not go to yoga because of not getting the handle of it quick enough or how their body is not built for yoga. Everyone struggles in the beginning, to get better is to practice. As an artist when I first started drawing it was not the best. As I continued and practiced more and more, I slowly got better, it goes the same for yoga. It is never an easy road, it can be longer for others and jerky for some but at the end, we all get to our destination.

Interview with Chelsea Roberts

Dr. Chelsea Jackson Roberts is a big influence in my life and I have been blessed to interview her. I wanted to see how she views yoga and get to know more on how it influence her life.

Where did you go to college, how many years?

BA - Spelman College - 4 years

MA - Teachers College, Columbia University - 2 years

PhD - Emory University - 5 years

Where do you work?

"Technically, I work around the globe as I travel leading workshops, conferences, and trainings for yoga teachers and educators. I am the co-founder of Red Clay Yoga and founder of Chelsea Loves Yoga."

What inspired you to do the Yoga Literature and Art camp?

"I started Yoga, Literature, and Art Camp because I used to be a teacher and I learned from my students more than anyone that movement, breathing, and feeling connected was essential when it came to learning. After I taught elementary school for 8 years, I decided to research the impact yoga has on learning. I decided to create a case study that later developed into YLA Camp! We are now going into our 5th year of the camp."

What is your personal experience with yoga and it's healing process?

"My experience with yoga and the healing process is that I can use the tools I learn in yoga (i.e., the breath, slowing down, and listening to my body) to understand what my body needs and what needs to be healed. I am learning everyday that the healing process, whether it is physical or emotional takes time. I love my yoga practice because it reminds me that time is all I have."

Is there any inspiration to doing what you do?

"My inspiration comes a lot from the youth (like you) with whom I work. When I see the excitement or peace that happens during a practice, I am inspired to continue to practice too. It reminds me that I am alive and our world is in good hands because the youth are learning more about themselves and others early. I see this happening through yoga."

What are your tips for beginners?

"My tips for beginners would simply be patience and exploration. Just notice the urge to compare your body to others, or your practice. Notice how it makes you feel when you do that. For me, not very good. Remember that yoga is not about sticking the perfect pose or knowing how to do a handstand. Yoga is being present with what is, and what is - is you and that is beautiful."

Do you believe there is a self (spiritual) awareness in meditation?

"I believe that everyone's yoga practice is unique to them. For me, yoga has definitely moved me deeper into my spiritual connections with the earth, with my Source, and within my relationships with others."

What are some of the struggles and benefits going into the yoga industry?

"For me, because I am both African American and I am a woman, it is a challenge to feel heard or seen at times. The "yoga industry"is very different than yoga the practice. The yoga industry thrives from selling products, trainings, conferences, retreats, and workshops; this can be a challenge because yoga should be accessed by all if there is an interest. Unfortunately, not everyone has access and not everyone is valued when it comes to advertising who yoga is for.

As far as benefits, I love what I do. I feel incredibly lucky and blessed to be able to practice yoga in some way, shape, or form everyday for my actual job. The people I meet as a result has been the biggest benefit for me."

Sanskrits (Yoga poses)

Yoga is full of many wonderful poses and postures that are profitable to the body and increase your range of movement and flexibility. There are many difficult poses in yoga, so I will be going over the basics. Yoga postures are already complex by itself, so breaking it into different sections will help to learn about them more straightforward. Each pose can have modifications to it if it means using a block for support or a pose modification.

Stomach-

Dhanurasana

Bow pose, or Dhanurasana, Dhanu meaning bow. It is called bow because it resembles an archer bow. It has many benefits including helping constipation, respiratory ailments, mild backache, fatigues, anxiety, and menstrual discomfort. Many find it hard to lift their thighs above the floor, to help support the thighs make sure to have a rolled blanket underneath both legs.

Setu Bandha Sarvangasana

The bridge pose is called Setu Bandha Sarvangasana, Setu meaning bridge and Bandha meaning lock. This pose holds many benefits including stretching the chest, neck, and spine. It relieves stress and mild depression. Physical benefits include improving digestion, helping menopause, relieving back aches, asthma, and many more. When you roll back the shoulders, make positive that you are not pulling them uncomfortably away from the ears. This tends to overstretch the neck bone. It avoids discomfort, lift your shoulders slightly nearing the ears and push the inner shoulders away from the spine.

Baddha konasana

Baddha konasana has many benefits for the body. Buddha meaning bound and Kona meaning angle. It is often difficult to get into the pose with lowered knees and a straighten back. To fix your posture, sit on an elevated surface. This pose helps prompt the abdominal organs, ovaries and prostate gland, bladder, and kidneys. It has great mental benefits such as fatigues and anxiety. Along with physical benefits such as circulation of the body, and stretches the inner thighs, groins, and kneecaps. Most of the benefits though correlate with the female body. Relieving symptoms of menopause, menstrual discomfort, and even childbirth.

Arms:

Bakasana

Crane pose (also known as crow pose) is named after its original name Bakasana, Baka meaning crane. Crane pose is a more challenging pose to do, even so, it gives assistance to the arms, abdominal muscles, wrist, and upper back. Many beginners have a tendency to raise with their backside far from their heels, which creates more struggle and an uncomfortable position. For more comfortability, try to keep yourself swaddled together with your heels and rear-end together. To push up in the air, use the support of the upper arms against the shins while drawing in your inner groins deep into the abdomen.

Gomukhasana

Go meaning cow and Mukha meaning face.

Cow face or Gomukhasana helps extend the shins, hips and upper thigh, shoulders, biceps and triceps, and chest area. Many people have much difficulty with getting their sitting bones to rest evenly on the floor, to fix this, grab a blanket or bolster and place underneath you. When the pelvis is tilted the spine won't be able to extend properly. It's a short pose with about twenty seconds on each side.

Astavakrasana

Astr meaning eight and vakra meaning bent or curved

  Eight angle pose or Astavakrasana helps strengthen the wrist and arms. This pose puts a great deal of pressure on the wrists and arms, and many beginners find it hard to balance in this pose. For support, what can help is putting a bolster underneath the hip and outer thigh.

Legs:

Parsvottanasana

Parsva meaning side, ut meaning intense, and tan meaning

stretch

Intense side stretch is a great pose for calming the brain, stretching the spine, shoulders, hips, and legs. Many people use this pose to help improve their posture and balance. Learners tend to lift their back heel up. To teach the foot to go back down, doing this pose with your back heel against a wall will force the foot to be grounded.

Padangusthasana

The big toe pose has similar benefits to the other ones but this one has a big benefit to fight insomnia and help the liver and kidneys. If it is hard to hold the toes without bending your knees, grabbing a yoga strap and hooking it to the sole of the foot will help deepen the stretch without breaking position.

Ardha Bhekasana

Half frog pose is profitable for those with high or low blood pressure, migraines, insomnia and low back/neck injuries. Bringing improvement of posture and stretches the entire front body. Many traditional texts say that the frog pose helps increases body heat and destroys diseases. For support, it is easier if the lower ribs have a bolster underneath.

Heart:

Utkatasana

utkata meaning powerful or fierce

Chair Pose or Utkatasana is great for lowering blood pressure. This pose helps with the ankles, thighs, calves, and spine. For assistance in this pose, doing this pose with your tailbone towards a wall makes this pose easier to get adjusted to. This pose helps stimulates the heart and abdominal muscles, along with fixing feet posture.

Bhujangasana

bhujanga meaning serpent

Cobra pose is a backbend pose, supporting the spine, chest, lungs, abdomen organs and heart. I found myself benefiting from this pose due to it releasing the stress and fatigues in my body. Therapeutic for people with asthma, it makes your lungs open up. Learners tend to overdo the backbend, straining the neck and back muscles. I recommend to not go beyond your limit and stay in a position you are comfortable with, all it does is hurt you more than it helps.

Kapotasana

King pigeon pose helps stretch the whole front body and lower part of the body. When bending over, it helps for novice learners are placing the crown of the head and feet towards the wall. This is an extreme version of pigeon pose, it is advised for people that are used to backbends and are more advanced to use this pose.

Lower Back:

Ardha Pincha Mayurasana

Dolphin pose is like downward facing dog, the difference is placing your forearms on the ground instead of the hands. The pose helps relieve stress and mild depression and help prevent osteoporosis. It is therapeutic for high blood pressure, asthma, flat feet, and sciatica. To help open the shoulders, lift the elbows on a rolled up sticky mat. While doing this, press the inner wrists against the floor.

Utthita Trikonasana

Triangle pose helps strengthens the thighs, knees, and ankles. Improving digestion, helping backaches, pregnancy, and relieving menopause. It is also very therapeutic for anxiety, infertility, neck pain, osteoporosis, and sciatica. If you feel unsteady in this pose, put your back heel against a wall.

Malasana

Garland pose, stretches the lower legs and back while also toning the torso. If squatting in this pose becomes difficult, sitting on the front edge of a chair is beneficial. Leaning the torso forward between the legs will create the same stretch. If the heels cannot reach the floor, placing a blanket underneath is helpful.

Brain:

Nadi Shodhana Pranayama

This pose is considered a formal pose by itself, channel-cleaning breath is the most beneficial to the mental part of yoga. Physical properties such as lowering the heart rate and reduces stress and anxiety. In meditation, it is said that this position helps synchronize the two hemispheres of the brain. Also, it is said to help purify the energy channels or nadis of the body so that the flow of prana is smoother during the practice. This is a form of meditation, to help the concentration in the mind, it is best to recite madras or focusing on an image or word.

Balasana

Many people do not believe that child's pose has any type of beneficial favours towards the body but as a breather in between intense poses. While it is a restorative pose, this position holds the support of a backbend. Lightly stretches the leg area and relieves back and neck pain. Breathing consciously in this backbend is vital in this pose. When exhaling in this pose, push the torso deeper into the fold almost like Marjariasana or cat pose.

Marichyasana I

Pose Dedicated to the Sage Marichi I is a great pose for

relaxing the mind, stretching the shoulder and spine area, and improving digestion. Many beginners have a hard time keeping the bent knee close to the torso. Which creates a troublesome strain to adjust the shin into the armpit and hug the arm around the leg. When you put the arm forward, in the beginning, grip the knee with the opposite-side hand. It will pull the thigh into the torso.

Singing Bowl healing

The sound is one important aspect of yoga. To bathe the senses with the enriching sounds of the singing bowl, it allows healing in the body. It really is an experience that everyone needs to have at least once in their life. This healing process is connected to the brain, intervening with the brain waves and creating a sense of calmness helps slowly heal the mind. When practiced, it shows to lower the activity of stress disorders, pain, and depression; this is a beneficial for those with stress related issues. This healing wonder has shown to heal people not only mentally but physically. Let's begin with the healing process.

Physical benefits

Sound therapy has been proven to help those with diseases like Cancer. The sonic waves that you hear awaken many parts of your brain, you can also feel the sound vibrations through your entire physical body. Many diseases are due to an imbalance of the cells in your body. Matter is energy vibrating at multiple rates, by changing the structure of matter by changing the speed of the vibration. With sound therapy such as singing bowls, the sound makes the Theta brain frequencies create a peaceful state. The vibrations have an impact on the nervous system, it makes the nervous system response with relaxation and peace. This is very beneficial to illnesses that have an imbalance with the vibrations in matter, which includes cancer. An article from the mindful word states,

[3]"Dr. Mitchell Gaynor has been using sound, including Tibetan bowls, crystal bowls and chanting in work with cancer patients for many years. The medical director of the Deepak Chopra Center in California, Dr. David Simon, found that the sound from Tibetan bowls as well as chanting are chemically metabolized into 'endogenous opiates' that act on the body as internal painkillers and healing agents."

[3] Writer, Contributing. "TIBETAN SINGING BOWLS: Introduction to sound healing with Tibetan Singing Bowls." The Mindful Word, 2 Apr. 2014, www.themindfulword.org/2011/tibetan-singing-bowls-introduction/.

With this in mind, imagine that every body part is vibrating at a different speed. With an imbalanced area of vibration, sound therapy will help resonate and restore each part of the body. Vibration dis-harmony in the muscles and the Alpha and Theta brainwave frequencies is some of the many difficulties that can be solved with using sound therapy.Sound therapy creates a reduction in brain wave activity. It alsos lowers the heart and respiratory rate, this creates something called "Cardio-Respiratory Synchronicity". This helps release blocked energy, while brining the body back into alignment.

Mental benefits

Along with physical benefits, it shows to have improvement on the mental and spiritual state. Many medical schools have even used this type of medical treatment to find incredible results in cancer patients. The program that links the mind body and spirit together is what universities like Duke and North Carolina have been using. There is founded spiritual awakening and a regenerative process to this type of therapy. Positive or negative attitudes and behaviors have an effect on our healing potential. Positive affirmations and visualization along with the sound vibration of the bowls, is a greatly enhance healing movement. Sound therapy as we know it is a type of energy medicine. Energy medicine, therapy, and healing are part of a branch in alternative medicine. Based on a belief that is pseudo-scientific, the healer can channel healing energy into a patient. This creates a spiritual area in which one can find rehabilitation or healing with stress disorders and depression. People with sleep disorders, PTSD, and pain management also are benefited by doing this. The healing process entertains your brainwaves with the vibrations in the bowl, it truly resonates with you.

Chakra healing

Many people do not know where to start on when they may feel their chakras unbalanced. Unbalanced chakras can cause stress and anxiety, depression, and a feeling of being a tedious version of yourself. Balancing your chakras can help with these thing with, of course, the exceptions of mental illness and mood disorders. People that are new to chakra tuning should always start off with a simple chakra awareness meditation. This will help make the body more aware of the blockages of energy and where it is happening. When trying to work on your own chakras, it is best to get comfortable. Relax in a soothing calm atmosphere and allow the tones to be felt completely. Relaxing scents and other elements will help enhance the experience. From experience, restorative yoga and chakra balancing go hand in hand.Chakra balancing have many different techniques and each person has their own way of fixing their own chakras. It is vital to experiment and try the one that works with you. With the typical visual, audible, and kinesthetic learners, it is the same with meditation. Many prefer to sing along with the bowel, due to having a hard time with visualization. While others tend to massage the palms of the hands, while concentration on each chakra. The beauty of this is that there is no incorrect way of balancing your chakras because it is what the individual sees fit. As long as there is a motivation to heal each one and love present, the meditation will work to many different people. To exfoliate the experience even more, refreshing what your intention is, mantras or prayers in the beginning may help set a tone. If there is a specific chakra you are working on then visualizing the energy center with brightness, the colour. Think about where is it placed, is it glowing, the size, and almost anything that can give you a visual representation of the chakra that you are focusing on. The chakra balancing is to refill love into the center. Using positive affirmations and mantras for the chakra and visualization of the love will help contribute to the overall beneficial ending. You can also do a "tune-up", refreshing all chakras. Starting from what many would call the base, or root chakra and working all the way up to the crown then back down. This will create an overall peace to the chakras. Even after meditation on one chakra, you can always check up on the rest of the chakra.

Environmental sounds

Our average day includes so many harsh and loud sounds and depending on where you live, it's harsher than others. These sounds can elevate our stress levels and make an imbalance in our nervous system. Living like this for a long enough time can create a decrease in our immunity and rare cases, hearing loss. Stress has a vital role in what we hear and how it affects us, with anxiety everyday sounds can become harsher and louder. With sound therapy, we can lower these affects, become better listeners and take awareness into the noises we absorbed. Just like healthy eating for the body to strengthen, healthy hearing to strengthen the ears. These practices can make us feel more grounded and centered. Sound is a source for inner peace in the bustling world of stress.

Certainly sound therapy is not a necessity, rather a optional privilege. Fortunitionaly, sound therapy with the connection of yoga is becoming more aware by modern medicine. Remember, your mind, spirit, and body is a working machine, so it is always beneficial to check it over for repairs. The experience I had with tibetan sound bowls was the first time I ever felt self-awareness. It truly is a privilege to experience this first handed, opening not only my senses but also my passion for yoga and meditation.

The Yoga Sūtras of Patañjali

The fundamentals of yoga belong to the Yoga Sūtras of Patañjali, where there is 196 sutras divided into four chapters or books. It is the foundation to the raja yoga system along with various kinds of awareness to the mind body and soul. It shows the eight holded path to yoga and the system to maintain the goal to liberation. This is the original key guide of yoga, it goes into detail of everything dealing with yoga and meditation. These are the guidelines to living a deep and meaningful life and has answered many puzzling questions about yoga. I will be going over each chapter and what each Pada beholds.

Samadhi Pada (51 sutras)

This chapter is about enlightenment and defining yoga as a whole along with the problems many face when doing yoga. The chapter focuses on the various kinds of samadhi along with the focus on different classifications. Original Sanskrit definition of Yoga is called Yoga Chitta Vritti Nirodha. Meaning to still the mind in order to achieve ultimate reality and block the modifications of consciousness is yoga. It explains the two essential qualities for success, abhyasa and vairagya. Abhyasa meaning constant practice and repetition and vairagya, meaning detachment from a physical level and more into your spiritual inner soul. Multiple types of samadhi are classified along with the two areas of samadhi viz. Samadhi viz is on a religious aspect of yoga meaning the union with the lord, it can be used in your views of religion as well. One category is sabija meaning with seed, nirbija meaning without seed is the other. Sabija holds six kinds of viz, chapter one ends with clarifying seedless awareness. Nirbija is only activated when you block all the chitta vrittis. Chitta vrittis meaning mind chatter or commonly called monkey mind, which is the jumbled up thoughts in your head.

Sadhana Pada (55 sutras)

Chapter two focuses on more of the practice, also known as Sadhana. Along with the obstacles, or kleshas of Sadhana. There are various fruits of the practice, the first six parts out of eight of yoga discipline all have these fruits. Along with this are five kleshas that signify the importance to overcome these obstacles. They bind down the physical body and truly keep us away from reaching our full potential. The first one being avidya meaning ignorance, asmita meaning egoism or selfishness, raga meaning passion or attachment, dvesha meaning anger, and finally abhinivesha, the fear of death. The chapter goes into the solution of getting rid of these kleshas and many different theoretical applications for your yoga practice. The chapter goes into the paths of a yoga practice called Raja, this is a type of practice that focuses on the self and raises your self-confidence. It begins with the moral codes of conduct or yamas, it is made up of five kinds of viz. The first code is ahimsa, meaning no violence, satya meaning being truthful, asteya meaning no theft, brahmacharya meaning abstinence, and aparigraha which is lack of greed. This goes further into the inner disciplines, these five morals are called niyamas. Presented in this section is shauca meaning purity, which can mean both physical and mental. Santosha meaning contentment and tapas meaning austerity. Svadhyaya meaning study for example, the study of religious text, stories and their own moral code. Ishvarapranidhana is the last one, meaning devotion of god. The chapter shows more of the religious form of yoga, as well as how to breath, posture, and withdrawal from physical reality.

Vibhuti Pada (56 sutras)

The last two limbs of yoga that were not discussed in chapter two are explained here. The two being dhyana being meditation and samadhi being awareness. This goes into the introduction of the notion of samyama as being the concurrent practice for the last three yoga branches. The chapter shows the fundamental aspects of samyama. Along with the detailed description on what can be obtained by doing this practice. It can be practiced on objects, ideas, and thoughts. By meditating on the powers described in the chapter, are described to give knowledge of the future, previous births, of other people's thoughts, and even the solar system and stars. It even states on how you can achieve levitation and invisibility. Given, this is based on religion and spiritual beliefs and leading yoga teachers agree that these abilities are not possible by the laws of physics. Even so, there has been benefits to the mind due to the fact that the mind seems to be more flexible. Yoga by itself can help empower the mind and open the brain up to achieve inner peace.

Kaivalya Pada (34 sutras)

This chapter helps us clarify and explore deeper into the liberation of the mind and how we can achieved this long awaited liberation. Vansanas also known as samskaras are subtle mental impressions become clear in the mind, having karmic effects. Vasanas are to vanish when killing off the four factors practically hetu meaning cause, phala meaning effect, ashraya meaning support of experience, and alambana meaning object of experience. This happens so that citta or higher mind can be purified and reflect drashta and drishya. Drashta meaning the observer or witness and drishya meaning the observed or seen. This demonstrates how the soul is part of true nature and going towards pure consciousness. The last chapter ends in the definition of liberation or kaivalya. Kaivalya meaning the state where the qualities fuse with their cause, causing there being no need for purpose due to finding pure consciousness or purusha.

Aromas in meditation and yoga

Along with using sound bowls to interact with the sense of sound, we can also use our sense of smell to enrich our experience in yoga and meditation. Incense burners and essential oil diffusers are not only used to deepen your meditative state but also in holistic medicine. It can help in the treatment of a variety in disease and illness including cancer, asthma, heart disease, migraines, and more. This can explain how many of them have such a costly price, saving up for oils and buying testers are always great for people that want to get into them more. The majority of essential oils should not been applied to the skin and eaten, typically many do not have artificials that keep it safe which also contributes to the strong smell it gives. Experimenting is also very beneficial to those who do not know what oils to use, different oils work on different people. Some might use lavender to help stress and sleep while others will find the opposite effect on them. Slowly adapt to using oils in your practice not only to help your body adjust and become aware to the new awakening, but also to feel the properties and the power of these oils stronger to the sense of smell.

[4]There is multiple forms of diffusing oils and some might appeal more pleasant than others. Experimenting on how your body prefers to experience the scent with yoga and meditation is highly advised. Some may go towards the safe for skin oils to rub on your hands and temples, others might like a diffuser to smell the aroma in the air. There is no right way to smell and there is always positive encouragement in trying out different scents in multiple forms.

Diffusing scents

The love of being surrounded in a space where the aroma is completely acute to your senses, where in the moment of meditation you are more focused on the sense of area around you. Diffusion scents are mists that are sprayed around your area of yoga or meditation. There is

---

[4] Word of caution- Many oils have large amounts of harmful ingredients or high acidic levels, always be careful when handling oils. Keep them out of reach of small children, and consult your doctor if you are pregnant, nursing, taking prescription medication, or have a medical condition.

many machines that are used to diffuse oils, along with oil lamps. This form of scent therapy is a great way to feel surrounded in the fragrance that you love, while most being very cost friendly.

Purifying scents

To feel cleanse with aromas that open up your senses in an expression of freedom. This form of expressing aromas is to purify the air and clean any horrible toxins, fungus, and bacteria in the air. Many use different types of blends to clean and refresh the air,along with your yoga space, yoga mat, furniture, and clothes. Some are easy to make at home, using harsher oils should be left to a professional. Many oils like lavender, peppermint, to frankincense are all good to refresh your home and life. Using a diffuser, lamps, and safe for touch sprays are all ways you can purify your home and treasures.

Anointing scents

Having the physical touch to the scent can evoke a strong connection to the aroma provoking powerful healing properties. Mostly used in restorative yoga to boost the relaxing power over your body, it is also used before yoga and meditation as an infuser of energy and life. Using the oil on your joints, inner wrists, temples, and any of the placements of the chakras will support meditation like chakra healing and finding inner peace. This form of aroma therapy is popular due to easy transportation and comfortability. The most common and affordable ways to use this application is with roll on oils, many come with how to use with chakra and the listing of benefits.

One of the most common confusions when dealing with oils is what oils to use for what benefits. There is a wide variety of types of scents in the world of yoga and it is recommended to expert with not so common ones to find your most preferred scent. There is so many common ones that show great healing properties. Here I will explain are a few categories and oils that are beneficial.

Grounding

Grounding is a term that is to describe being connected to the now of things or present. Meaning to also follow life's purpose, to be productive, and focusing. Not being grounded can lead to disorganization, lack of sleep, scattered thought, and not being able to make affirmative decisions. It is to be connected to what's happening now, when you are feeling brain fog or dazed these are the oils you can turn to.

- **Ylang Ylang**- Ylang Ylang oil has many properties of an antidepressant and an antiseptic. It is great for immune health and blood circulation, making it a alternative medicine for cardiovascular, reproductive and digestive problications.

- **Frankincense**- Frankincense shows great benefits for mental health. Including reducing stress levels and mood swings, while preventing illness and strengthening your immune system. Helps fight cancer and chemotherapy side effects, killing harmful germs and healing the skin.

- **Cypress-** To heal cuts and open wounds quickly, appling cypress oil helps, along with other wounds and infections. Treating cramps and muscle pains along with many more physical properties. Also becoming a natural deodorant and relieves anxiety.

- **Cedarwood-** Improving focus and brain functionality, along with activating the brain with similarities like fish oil. Cedarwood is beneficial to your gums and teeth during toothaches, along with anti-inflammatory substances. Along with skin and hair healing properties it is great addition to your beauty routine.

- **Ginger-** Ginger is one of the more popular and common in the holistic medicine industry. Various stomach problems, side effects from cancer treatment, nausea caused by HIV and AIDS treatment, and after surgery vomiting are all cured by ginger.

Chakra healing

Chakra healing is vital to your mental tranquility and meditation practice. There are many different causes to chakra imbalance, the imbalanced system can interfere with everyday activities and decreases your overall productivity. When doing chakra healing meditation, to heal in meditation it is beneficial to use essential oils to enhance your practice. Using the right aromas can help open up the channels that energy flows through and each chakra.

- Root chakra

Patchouli oil has proven to be a great antidepressant and febrifuge, it is also a insecticide and fungicide. This is a tonic substance that will help make your body feel more grounded and aware of the present and lift any type of brain fog.

- Sacral chakra

Sandalwood is one of essential oils that create a calm and therapeutic scent that will help you achieve clarity. Feel many healing benefits to help your mental health and overall well-being, making this scent great for the sacral chakra.

- Solar Plexus Chakra

Cinnamon is a strong and great scent not only for heating up this chakra, but also for any physical health drawbacks that you want to see disappear. Many physical benefits include many anti-inflammatory abilities, helping the heart, and from fighting diabetes and cancer to dental health. Cinnamon can not only be used for chakra healing, but also much more.

- Heart chakra

Roses are known for their beautiful scent and aesthetically pleasing form, the more we study of this flower although, the more factors we can see that play a positive toll on the body. Roses are fully packed with vitamins, minerals, and like the above list of oils, anti-inflammatory benefits. Roses hold many uses for skin care, helping dry skin, treating redness, and acneic skin. It is used for the heart chakra due to it's symbol of love and mental benefits such as fighting depression and insomnia.

- Throat chakra

Eucalyptus is a more well-known and commonly used oil, due it being entirely colourless and and having a unique taste and smell. Eucalyptus is a holistic medicine popularity due to the wide-range of medical qualities. It is used as an antispasmodic, decongestant, antibacterial, and even in some deodorant. It is used in the throat chakra due to its healing properties of curing throat related illness and sinuses. This leads to having clear passageway to feel the freedom and self-expression that this chakra is suppose to be about.

- Third eye chakra

Lavender, being more common than Eucalyptus but also not as talked about outside being a stress reliever. It is able to reduce nervous tension, but it can also be a disinfect the scalp and the skin and a pain reliever. Lavender is a great treatment for the respiratory systems and improving the blood circulation.

- Crown chakra

Frankincense and Helichrysum oil are beneficial to the crown chakra, since I have talked about frankincense I will be going over Helichrysum oil and the benefits. Helichrysum oil is a great skincare treatment for those with sunburns, skin cancer, acne, and overall being a great antibiotic for your skin. While also being a great factor for your heart health and digestive and diuretic system.

Breathing

Having clear breath is vital in your health due to its relation to the lungs and throat. Clear breath will allow a deeper meditation and yoga experience. Relief, reconnecting, and rejuvenating are all experiences that you should feel in connecting with your breath.

Palo Santo

Palo Santo oil is used traditionally to treat common colds, the flu, asthma, and headaches. It is also shown to treat emotional pain and anxiety and depression. Not only is this a great essential oil for meditation, but it can also be used in the art of massage to also support the healing process.

Lemon (Citrus limon)

Despite lemons being very acidic, it can be very stimulating when used in meditation. It is used for anti-infection, but it can also be used for detoxifying and great for healing the body. It helps the throat open up and become clear.

Oregano

Oregano oil has many of the same benefits of the herb, full of antioxidants. Internal use for illness and external use for skin infections such as yeast infections are common uses for oregano. It is also stimulating for the immune system, which also leads to better breathing.

Thyme

A medicinal herb since the ancient era, being a very strong antioxidants. If you are feeling congested or having any infections in the chest or throat, thyme is the herb to turn to. It is great for clear breathing due to it's the to serenity the common cold, coughing, and throat infections.

Tea Tree

Tea tree oil is most commonly used for the skin and hair. It is great for skin infections such as acne and fungal infections in the nails. Hair treatments of tea tree oil is greatly used for lice, tea tree oil is also the remedy of athlete's foot and ringworm. This oil is great for opening up the lungs and sinuses in meditation.

Spiritual properties

1. Geranium

   Dealing with heaviness in the heart, sham for your actions, and overall a sharp pain in your spirit are overall occuring feelings in life. Geranium oil is a gentle yet powerful oil that will nourish your soul and heal the pains in your heart chakra. In chinese medicine, it is shown to enter the liver and kidneys, it is a deep and healing oil that is beneficial to the spirit. It is estrogenic though, use caution when having cysts or breast cancer. Even so, it brings great pleasure to those who uses it.

2. Pine

Pine oil has a strong yang core which is favorable to those with self loathing issues and create an energetic clearnese. It helps with clarity and support those who feel like they lost their purpose in life, pain, guilt, and breakups. Chinese medicine says how it enters the lungs and kidneys and is usually used with epsom salt. Supporting adrenals and giving energy to your kidneys.A small amount goes a long way, a few drops can show some clarity in life.

3. Rosemary

Low self esteem, lack of self-confidence, depression, and mental strain are only some of the things that make our spirit wilter and rattles us to a point of fatigueness if not stopped. Rosemary contains elements that help fight off these spiritual and mental difficulties. Rosemary oil works on many levels of the body from the skin to the memory, this oil has so many benefits that it can be used in any situation.

4. Yarra yarra

   Yarra yarra oil helps numerous skin problems along with bleeding, rashes, acne, dryness and many more. This oil destroys bacteria, fungus, and other types of microbes. The oil also has many tranquilizing properties, it can help the heart and calming the nerves. It is proven to help those with hypertension, insomnia, stress and the immune system.

Eucalyptus oils

There is over 700 species of eucalyptus oils in the world. It is confusing on what type to pick and many of them being overpriced and out of reach. Many label it under the label of Eucalyptus not understanding what it means and only parts of the plant being marketed, this can be very confusing. However, there is many types of oil that are commonly used and easy to apply. These next seven types of Eucalyptus oils are not only easy to find on the market, but also very beneficial to the body and mind.

Globulus- This oil is a more popular oil on the Eucalyptus market. It is a great treatment for upper respiratory infections because of this oil being a great decongestant alternative medicine. It is commonly used for the chest to heal fevers and colds. The oils is inhaled, which can soothe congestion and sore throats.

Radiata- This oil is represented to more gentle than the others, this means that it can be used almost at any age. This oil is very well-rounded in terms of beneficial properties to the body. This includes respiratory, multiple types of infections, aches and muscle pains, and even great for massage blend. Radiata oil is targeted to small children and the elderly due to its benefits in helping blood circulation and those with arthritis.

Dives - Also known as peppermint eucalyptus because of its unique minty smell. The strong smell makes this oil a great decongestant for those with chest colds and bronchitis. Dives are great for muscle pain and reducing it. Along with support with reducing fever and improving circulation, by increasing blood flow and reducing lung infections. Dives is a great antibacterial and anti-inflammatory alternative medicine.

Citriodora- also known as lemon eucalyptus is great for stopping mosquito, deer, and tick bites. It is also great for muscle spasms. Osteoarthritis, joint pain, and even toenail fungus or known as onychomycosis. The lemon scent makes it great for colds, relieves congestion, and can be used as a chest rub.

Eucalyptus Blue- This aroma that seems to be a fusion between Citriodora and globulus eucalyptus. It also does not cause reactions to allergies, which is why it is preferred. It is also has a higher preference than prescription medication due to it being an alternative seasonal allergy medicine. Along with sore muscles and infections.

Staigeriana- Staigeriana oil also known as lemon-scented Ironbark. For the skin, it is great for for wounds, burns, and bug bites. It also shoves off sluggish attitudes and stress from the mind. This oil is also a great inhalant and helps people with colds and prevents the spread of germs.

Different oils can be used in a multitude of ways, there is so many different reasons as well for someone to might use it. Oils hold many beneficial properties that goes back to ancient civilizations. Oils are traced to some great holistic medical properties and is greatly used among alternative medical professionals.

Children in yoga

Children have small attention spans, it can be hard to get their attention and to stay concentrated. It might be hard to focus them on academics or reading, but to many it seems impossible to get them into yoga. As a small child I have also struggled with concentration, I prefered high movement sports like swimming, soccer, and even kickboxing. Even so, I still struggled with anxiety and because of this I really tried to get into it. I went to hot yoga sessions with my mom and tried television yoga programs at home before I went to sleep. I struggled to get into it, but after awhile it starting transitioning into my daily routine and I got more adjusted to it. I also have a sister, she also has anxiety and quickly found a love for yoga when she was around the age of eleven. It is not impossible for kids to find a connection with yoga, but it can be very challenging. Many parents would love for their kids to get into yoga, I have spoke to many that don't know where to start. It starts out with baby steps and grows more and more into a fun experience for both parents and kids.

Getting your kid into yoga

Kids love chanting and humming, usually any type of sounds and interaction during yoga will help any kid stay engaged. Not only will it help them stay focused, but it will also make their meditation a more meaningful one. This builds a deep rooted connection with yoga for them and will make them see yoga as more than just an exercise. Blending in music in the background and bells will also get them engaged. Kids typically love to have an area for yoga then just doing it on the carpet in front of the television. Creating an area in your home for yoga will make them more motivated to do it. It can mean adding yoga mats and blankets, to making an alter in a corner of the kids room for meditation. Alters are not only used for religious rituals, in kids rooms it can be a fun and creative area where they can do yoga. It can be completely customizable where as they can add feathers, their favorite stuffed animals, or crystals.

This is a way to teach children gratitude will help ground the spirit. My alter is full of essential oils, stones, plants, and everything that I am grateful for.

Many children tend not to feel motivated when they are the only ones doing it, just like doing homework alone rather with friends. Yoga classes and sessions are great ways to get your kid to do yoga with other people their age, this way they will become more comfortable and accustomed to the practice. It can also make them gain friends along the way. Family yoga is also another way, because they are more comfortable with their family it will become a positive experience for them. The location of where you do your yoga and meditation is very important due to the experience it brings forth. Many people do not think about their environment when doing yoga, but imagine this, would you rather do yoga in a stuffy apartment or outside on a beach? It doesn't have to be as drastic, but creating a pleasant environment for your child will create a great feeling of accomplishment. Environment and setting affect children greater than adults, and it can make or break their yoga practice. Adding a nice background of plants or pictures, putting on meditative music, and even using aromas can help. When it's nice outside go to the park, go to yoga classes, and even an alter are all factors of helping your child get into yoga. All these things combined will really make the experience a more meaningful one, this is for all ages too.

Yoga has as many benefits in children as it does with adults and they need it as much too. There is many stressful factors in the lives of children that can be reduced through yoga. Physically, the benefits seem to be the same as in adults, flexibility, body awareness, coordination, and strength. It also has an enhancement on concentration for children along with relaxation and a sense of calm improves. Yoga for children is not only exercise and play but it can also bring a connection to a more deep inner self. It helps kids create a strong relationship with nature and the world around them. Yoga helps children mentally in getting back on track with school, friends and family. Yoga can be therapeutic to all ages.